What's Really in your Dog's Bowl?

The Essential Guide to Natural Nutrition.

By Majella Gee

Copyright © 2024 by Majella Gee. All rights reserved.

No part of this book may be reproduced, distributed, or transmitted in any form or by any means, including photocopying, recording, or other electronic or mechanical methods, without the prior written permission of the publisher, except in the case of brief quotations embodied in critical reviews and certain other non-commercial uses permitted by copyright law. For permission requests, write to the publisher, addressed "Attention: Permissions Coordinator," at the address below.

Publisher Contact Information:
Sorjam Publishing
Email: hello@majellaspetstore.com
Website: https://majellaspetstore.com/

This book is a work of nonfiction. The author has made every effort to ensure the accuracy and completeness of the information contained herein. However, the author and publisher assume no responsibility for errors, omissions, or any consequences arising from the use of this material.

Disclaimer:
The information provided in this book is intended for educational purposes and is not a substitute for professional veterinary advice. Always consult with a qualified veterinarian before making any significant changes to your pet's diet or lifestyle. The author and publisher disclaim any liability arising directly or indirectly from the use of this book.

ISBN: 978-1-7636631-1-4

Dedication

To every animal that has walked, flown, or crawled
into my life,
you have been my greatest teachers.
Through your trust, resilience, and spirit,
you've shown me the true meaning of compassion.
This book is for you—
for the lessons you've taught me
and the knowledge I now share with others,
in the hope that all animals can live happier,
healthier lives.

Acknowledgments

To all the animals who have come into my life, each one unique, each with their own lessons to teach. Like children, no two have ever been the same, and I've learned to listen closely to what they need. From those with allergies and sensitivities to those who thrived with ease, you've all shaped my understanding of true care.

To the specialized veterinarians and professionals, I've worked alongside, thank you for sharing your knowledge and your passion for animal welfare. Our collaborations have deepened my understanding, and I am forever grateful for the insights gained from working with some of the best in the field.

But most of all, to the animals themselves—thank you for your trust. You have taught me more than any book or classroom ever could. Through your behaviour, your needs, and your resilience, you've shown me how to listen. This book is for you, and I hope it helps others learn to hear what you're telling us.

Table of Contents

1. **Introduction**
   - The Truth About Commercial Pet Food – Time to Wake Up
2. **Chapter 1: Raw & Natural Diets for Dogs—Life Stage-Specific Diet Plans**
   - Components of a Balanced Raw Diet
   - The Great Garlic Debate
   - Bones: Types, Benefits, and Safety
   - Feeding Puppies: Growth and Vitality
   - Adult Dogs: Sustaining Energy and Health
   - Seniors: Supporting Joint Health and Digestion
3. **Chapter 2: Recipes for Specific Health Conditions**
   - Joint Health & Arthritis
   - Skin Allergies
   - Weight Management
   - Digestive Health
4. **Chapter 3: Hydration and Its Importance**
   - Clean Water vs. Tap Water
   - Hydrating Foods
   - Signs of Dehydration in Dogs
5. **Chapter 4: Monitoring Your Dog's Health Through Diet**
   - Understanding Your Dog's Poop (Yes, It Matters!)
   - Coat Condition and Energy Levels
   - How Behaviour Can Reflect Diet
6. **Chapter 5: Saving on Vet Bills—How a Natural Diet Keeps Your Dog Healthy**
   - Preventing Common Health Issues
   - Long-Term Savings from Feeding Real Food
   - A Healthier, Happier Dog
7. **Chapter 6: Putting It All Together—Recipes for Every Life Stage and Condition**
   - Key Puppy Recipes

- - Key Adult Dog Recipes
  - Key Senior Dog Recipes
  - Customising for Specific Health Needs
8. **Chapter 7: Bonus Recipes—Treats for Every Occasion**
    - Pocket Snacks for Walks
    - Moist Treats for Older Dogs
    - Icy Treats for Summer
    - Weight-Loss Treats
    - Fun Holiday and Birthday Treats
    - Global Treats for Specific Breeds
9. **Chapter 8: The 30-Day Transition to Nutrition Challenge**
    - Week 1: 25% Natural Foods
    - Week 2: 50% Natural Foods
    - Week 3: 75% Natural Foods
    - Week 4: 100% Natural Diet
    - What to Expect After 30 Days
    - Keeping the Momentum Going
    - Share Your Journey with #TransitionToNutrition
10. **Call to Action: Join the Natural Dog Nutrition Revolution!**
    - Share Your Journey
    - Visit Our Website
    - Exclusive Discount
    - Leave a Review
11. **Glossary**
    - Key Nutritional Terms
    - Harmful Additives in Commercial Dog Food
    - Beneficial Ingredients for a Natural Diet
12. **About the Author**
13. **Legal Notice**

Introduction

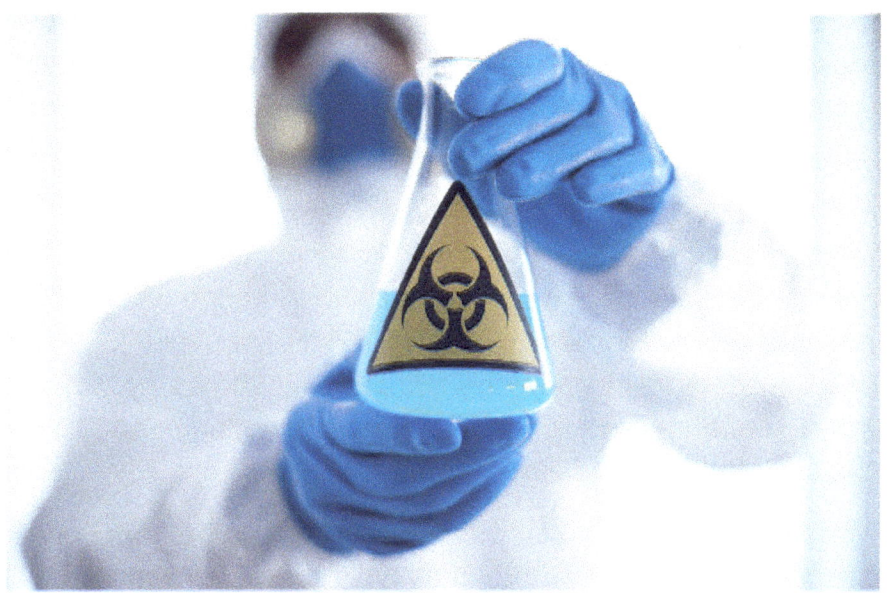

The Truth About Commercial Pet Food—Time to Wake Up

When it comes to feeding our pets, most of us have been led to trust the commercial pet food industry without much question. We see labels claiming, "complete nutrition" or "vet-approved," and we assume we're doing the best for our dogs. But it's time to wake up. The truth is, many of the commercial foods we feed our pets are full of harmful ingredients—preservatives, fillers, and synthetic chemicals that can lead to long-term health problems like cancer, obesity, diabetes, and joint pain.

Think about it: when was the last time you saw a wolf in the wild with obesity or arthritis? Wild animals don't suffer from the same chronic health issues our pets do. Why? Because they're eating a natural diet, free from the processed junk that fills so many commercial pet foods.

It's not just what's in the food—it's also what our pets are exposed to in their daily environments. From chemicals in the home (air fresheners, carpet cleaners, etc.) to the medications and treatments we're encouraged to use, our pets are bombarded with toxins. Add a diet of over-processed, nutrient-poor kibble to the mix, and it's no wonder they're suffering from allergies, tumours, joint pain, and behavioural issues.

My journey into understanding pet nutrition came from years of observing animals—both in the wild and in homes—and seeing the direct impact that poor diets and toxic environments have on their health. I've witnessed firsthand the tragic consequences of trusting what the pet food industry sells us as "healthy." Too many animals are suffering needlessly, and it's time to take responsibility as pet owners.

In this book, we're going to strip away the marketing myths and get back to basics. Feeding our pets shouldn't be complicated, but it does require us to ask questions, read labels, and make more informed choices. Our dogs rely on us to make decisions that will give them the best chance for a long, healthy life.

The solution? A raw, natural diet. It's time to move away from processed foods and embrace what nature intended. By feeding our pets whole, real foods, we can support their health in ways that commercial foods simply can't. This book will provide you with everything you need to start that journey—life stage-specific meal plans, recipes for specific health conditions, hydration tips, and much more.

Let's wake up, take action, and give our dogs the nutrition they deserve. They depend on us to keep them healthy, and that starts with what we put in their bowls.

Chapter One

Raw & Natural Diets for Dogs—Life Stage-Specific Diet Plans

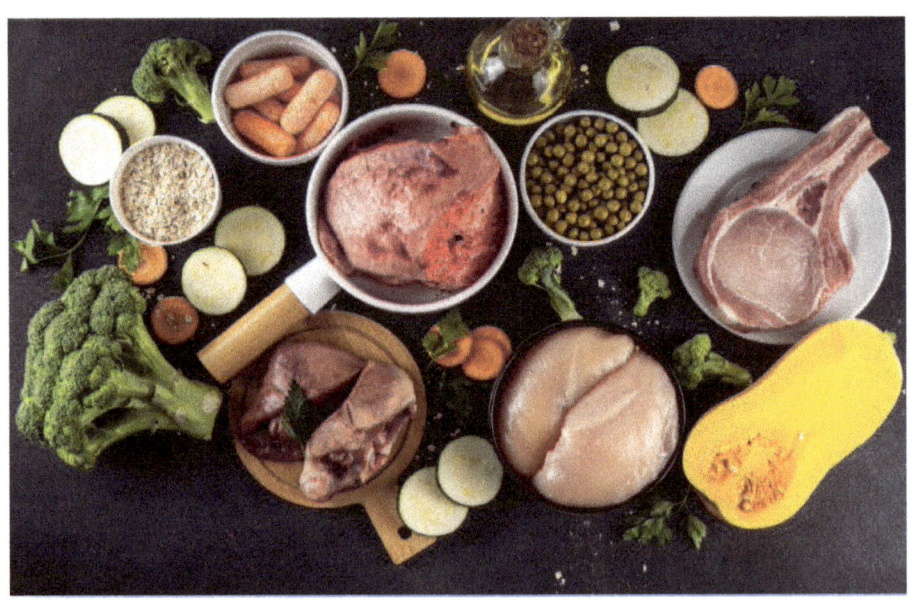

Introduction: Feeding Your Dog Like Nature Intended

A dog's nutritional needs change throughout their life—from the rapid growth of a puppy to the maintenance required during adulthood, and finally, the support needed during their senior years. A natural diet mimics what wild canines eat, ensuring your dog thrives at every life stage.

This chapter breaks down the essential dietary needs for puppies, adults, and seniors, offering one key recipe for each stage. These recipes are designed to provide balanced nutrition with whole, unprocessed foods, free from fillers and additives. For those looking to explore more meal options, be sure to check out the **Bonus Recipe Section** at the end of the book.

Components of a Balanced Raw Diet

A balanced raw diet includes a variety of components that contribute to a dog's overall health and well-being. Here's a breakdown of each element and how it supports a dog's natural nutritional needs:

1. **Protein Sources**
   Protein is the foundation of a dog's diet, providing essential amino acids for muscle health, energy, and cell repair. Common protein sources include chicken, beef, lamb, and fish, all of which are highly bioavailable and align well with a dog's carnivorous needs.
2. **Offal (Organ Meats)**
   Offal, or organ meats, is nature's multivitamin, packed with nutrients not found in muscle meat alone. Here are some key types of offal and their benefits:
   - **Liver**: High in vitamin A, iron, and folate, liver supports immune health, vision, and skin.
   - **Kidney**: Rich in B vitamins, iron, and selenium, which support metabolism and kidney health.
   - **Heart**: Contains taurine and CoQ10, beneficial for cardiovascular health and cellular function.

For a balanced diet, offal should make up around 5-10% of the total diet, with variety to avoid nutrient overload. Rotate organ meats like liver, kidney, and heart to ensure a balanced intake of essential vitamins and minerals.

3. **Raw Vegetables and Fruits**
   Although dogs don't need a large amount of plant-based food, a small portion of vegetables and fruits can provide fibre, vitamins, and antioxidants. Vegetables are best blended or pureed to aid in digestion, mimicking the partially digested plant matter dogs would consume in prey animals.
   - **Leafy Greens**: Spinach, kale, and parsley provide iron, calcium, and antioxidants.
   - **Root Vegetables**: Carrots and sweet potatoes are rich in beta-carotene and fibre.
   - **Preparation Method**: Blending vegetables with a small amount of offal can enhance nutrient absorption. Vegetables should make up no more than 10% of the diet.

The Great Garlic Debate: A Balanced Perspective

You've probably heard garlic is toxic to pets, but here's the truth—it depends on how it's used. While large amounts of garlic can be harmful, moderate amounts can actually benefit dogs.

Why I Use Garlic for My Dogs

When fed correctly, garlic offers incredible health benefits:

- **Flea and Tick Prevention:** Adding garlic to your dog's diet twice a week makes them less appealing to pests.
- **Immune Support:** Garlic contains antioxidants that strengthen the immune system.
- **Heart Health:** It supports healthy blood pressure and circulation.

How to Use Garlic Safely

- **Frequency:** Feed garlic twice a week as a natural flea and tick deterrent.
- **Dosage:**
    - Small dogs (up to 5kg): ¼ clove.
    - Medium dogs (6–15kg): ½ clove.
    - Large dogs (16–30kg): 1 clove.
    - Giant dogs (31kg+): 1½ cloves.
- **Preparation:** Crush or chop garlic and let it sit for 10 minutes to activate its beneficial compounds.

Important Note: Garlic is not safe for cats and should never be given to them. If your dog has pre-existing health conditions, consult your vet first.

Bones: Types, Benefits, and Safety

Bones are a crucial component of a raw diet, providing essential minerals, dental health benefits, and mental stimulation. Here's a closer look at the types of bones, their nutritional benefits, and guidelines for safe feeding.

1. **Types of Bones:**
    - **Meaty Bones:** These are bones with a good amount of meat still attached, such as chicken

wings, turkey necks, and lamb ribs. Meaty bones are softer and provide both nutritional benefits and dental health support.
    - **Recreational Bones**: Larger, harder bones like beef knuckles are primarily for chewing and mental enrichment. While they don't provide significant nutritional benefits, they help keep teeth clean and satisfy your dog's chewing instincts.
2. **Nutritional Benefits**:
    - Bones are a natural source of **calcium and phosphorus**, which are vital for strong bones and teeth.
    - **Bone marrow** contains fat and essential nutrients that contribute to a dog's energy needs and support immune health.
3. **Safety Guidelines**:
    - **Always feed bones raw**: Cooked bones can splinter, posing a choking hazard or causing digestive issues.
    - **Choose bone size carefully**: Match the bone size to your dog's size and chewing habits to avoid choking.
    - **Supervise while feeding**: Monitor your dog when they're chewing bones to ensure they are safe and not attempting to swallow bones whole.

Feeding bones can support dental health and mental stimulation, while also delivering essential minerals that contribute to a balanced, natural diet. Introducing bones gradually and observing your dog's chewing behaviour can ensure a safe and beneficial experience.

Feeding Puppies: Growth and Vitality

Puppies are growing rapidly, and they need nutrient-dense food that provides them with the essential building blocks for strong bones, muscles, and a healthy immune system. A diet rich in high-quality protein, healthy fats, and vitamins is crucial for this stage.

Key Nutrients for Puppies:

- **Proteins**: Choose easily digestible proteins like chicken, turkey, and lamb.
- **Offal (Organ Meats)**: Introducing offal, such as liver or heart, provides crucial vitamins (A, B) and minerals like iron, which are essential for healthy blood and immune development.
- **Bones**: Include softer, raw bones like chicken necks or wings to support dental health and provide essential calcium. Puppies benefit from raw bones as a natural source of nutrients for strong bone growth.
- **Vegetables**: Blended leafy greens, such as spinach and kale, provide fibre and vitamins. Blending or pureeing these vegetables helps puppies digest and absorb their nutrients better.

Key Puppy Recipe: Raw Chicken & Veggie Mash

Ingredients:

- 1 cup ground chicken (or turkey)
- ½ cup shredded carrots
- ¼ cup pumpkin puree
- 1 tablespoon coconut oil
- 1 small portion (approx. 1-2 teaspoons) raw liver (chicken or beef)

Instructions:
Mix all ingredients together and serve fresh. This recipe provides puppies with protein for growth, essential vitamins from vegetables, and healthy fats to support brain development. The addition of raw liver offers crucial vitamins A and B, which are beneficial for immune health and overall vitality. The pumpkin aids digestion, making this meal easy on a puppy's stomach.

Tip: Rotate proteins (chicken, turkey, beef) throughout the week to ensure your puppy gets a variety of nutrients, supporting balanced growth and health.

Feeding Adult Dogs: Sustaining Energy and Health

Once your dog reaches adulthood, their energy needs level out, but they still require a balanced diet to maintain their muscles, energy levels, and coat health. The focus should be on lean proteins, healthy fats, and fibre-rich vegetables to promote digestion and overall well-being.

Key Nutrients for Adults:

- **Proteins**: Incorporate a variety of meats, such as chicken, beef, and lamb, to provide a full range of amino acids.
- **Offal (Organ Meats)**: Rotate through organ meats like kidney and heart to supply taurine, B vitamins, and minerals such as zinc. These nutrients support cardiovascular health, immunity, and skin.
- **Bones**: Include meaty bones, such as turkey necks or lamb ribs, as a natural source of

calcium and phosphorus. Chewing on raw bones also keeps teeth clean and satisfies a dog's natural chewing instincts.
- **Vegetables**: Carrots, sweet potatoes, and kale offer additional fibre and antioxidants, supporting digestion and immune function.

Key Adult Dog Recipe: Beef & Sweet Potato Stew

Ingredients:

- 1 cup lean beef, cubed
- ½ cup sweet potatoes, chopped (lightly steamed if necessary)
- ¼ cup green beans, chopped (optional to steam)
- 1 small portion (approx. 1-2 tablespoons) raw liver or kidney
- 1 teaspoon fish oil (rich in omega-3s)

Instructions:

Mix the raw beef and liver or kidney with sweet potatoes and green beans. For easier digestion, lightly steam the sweet potatoes and green beans, if needed, but leave the meats raw for maximum nutrient retention. Add fish oil before serving to support joint health and a healthy coat. The inclusion of offal enhances the meal with vital vitamins and minerals.

Tip: Rotate the type of offal (liver or kidney) weekly for balanced nutrient intake. Also, try swapping green beans with other vegetables, like spinach or carrots, for added fibre and antioxidants.

Feeding Senior Dogs: Supporting Joint Health and Digestion

As dogs age, their metabolism slows, and they may experience joint stiffness or digestive sensitivities. A diet rich in lean, easily digestible proteins, anti-inflammatory ingredients, and joint-supporting supplements like glucosamine can help seniors stay healthy and comfortable.

Key Nutrients for Seniors:

- **Proteins**: Opt for leaner meats, like turkey or fish, which are easier on digestion and provide anti-inflammatory omega-3s.
- **Offal (Organ Meats)**: Increase liver and heart intake slightly for omega-3 fatty acids, which are anti-inflammatory and help support joint health. These also help maintain cognitive function and overall vitality in older dogs.
- **Bones**: Provide softer bones or reduce bone portions to ease digestion while still delivering calcium. Larger, dense bones may be harder to chew and digest for seniors.
- **Vegetables**: Blended greens, broccoli, and small portions of root vegetables offer antioxidants and fibre, supporting digestion and immune health.

Key Senior Dog Recipe: Chicken & Bone Broth Soup

- 1 cup shredded chicken (raw or lightly cooked if needed)
- ½ cup bone broth (rich in glucosamine and chondroitin)

- ¼ cup pumpkin puree
- 1 small portion (approx. 1-2 teaspoons) raw liver or heart (optional)
- 1 teaspoon turmeric (anti-inflammatory)

Instructions:

Combine the shredded chicken, bone broth, and optional raw liver or heart. Stir in the pumpkin puree and turmeric. Serve warm or at room temperature. This soup provides joint support through bone broth and turmeric, while the chicken and pumpkin offer easily digestible protein and fibre. The addition of offal adds essential vitamins and minerals beneficial for immune health and cognitive function in older dogs.

Tip: Bone broth is an excellent source of joint-supporting nutrients; make sure to use low-sodium varieties if store-bought or make your own at home for maximum benefits. Rotate different offal types to give a balanced intake of nutrients.

Conclusion: Adjusting the Diet for Every Life Stage

As your dog grows from puppy to adult and into their senior years, their dietary needs will evolve. A balanced, whole-food diet ensures they stay healthy and vibrant at every stage of life. The key is to adjust the proportions of nutrients—more protein and fats for puppies, fibre and antioxidants for adults, and joint support and easy-to-digest foods for seniors.

For even more meal ideas, head to the **Bonus Recipe Section** at the back of this book. There, you'll find a variety of fun and nutritious recipes to keep your dog happy and healthy, no matter their age or condition.

Chapter Two

Recipes for Specific Health Conditions

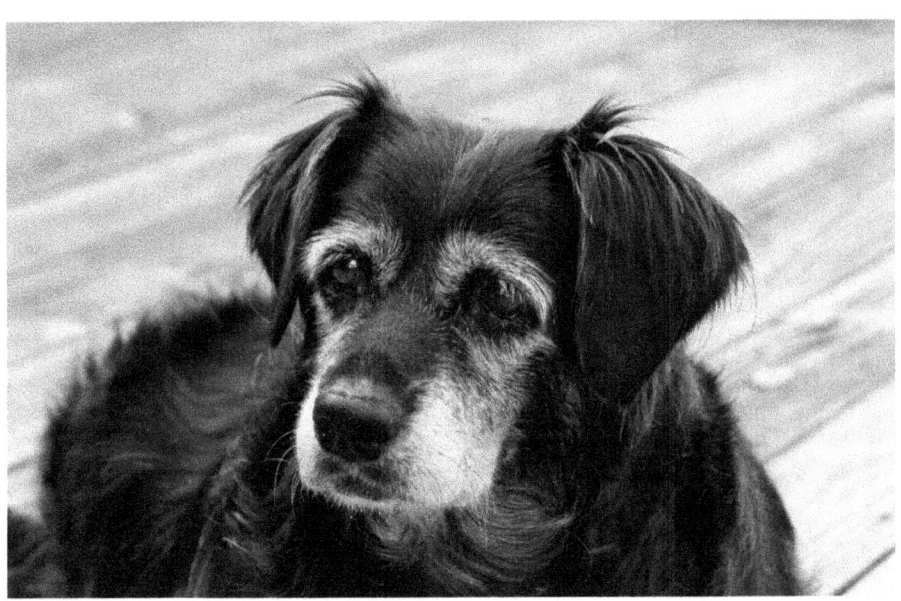

Introduction: Tailoring Diets for Special Needs

Dogs, like humans, can experience various health conditions that require special dietary adjustments. A natural, whole-food diet provides a solid foundation, but sometimes specific health issues need targeted nutritional support. Whether your dog is struggling with joint pain, allergies, weight management, or digestive issues, the right food can make a significant difference.

This chapter covers common conditions and provides **two recipes per ailment**, offering a variety of options to help support your dog's health.

---

1. Joint Health & Arthritis

As dogs age, joint pain and arthritis can become a common issue. Foods rich in **omega-3 fatty acids, glucosamine,** and **anti-inflammatory ingredients** like **turmeric** can help reduce pain and inflammation while supporting joint health.

Recipe 1: Bone Broth & Turkey Stew

Ingredients

- 1 cup shredded turkey (raw or lightly cooked if preferred)
- ½ cup bone broth (homemade or low sodium)
- ¼ cup green beans, chopped (optional to steam)
- 1 teaspoon fish oil
- 1 teaspoon turmeric
- 1 small portion (approx. 1 tablespoon) raw liver or kidney (optional for added vitamins and minerals)

Instructions:

Combine the raw or lightly cooked turkey with the bone broth, green beans, and optional raw liver or kidney. Stir in the fish oil and turmeric just before serving. Bone broth provides glucosamine for joint support, and turmeric and fish oil help reduce inflammation. The optional offal enhances the nutrient profile with essential vitamins and minerals for joint and immune health.

Recipe 2: Sardine & Sweet Potato Mash

Ingredients

- 1 can sardines (in water, no added salt)
- ½ cup mashed sweet potatoes (optional to lightly steam)
- ¼ cup spinach, chopped (optional to steam lightly)
- 1 teaspoon flaxseed oil (rich in omega-3s)
- 1 small portion (approx. 1-2 teaspoons) raw liver or kidney (optional for nutrient boost)

Instructions:

Mash the sardines and mix with sweet potatoes, spinach, and optional raw liver or kidney. Drizzle with flaxseed oil before serving. Sardines and flaxseed oil are high in omega-3s to reduce inflammation, while sweet potatoes provide fibre and vitamins. Adding offal boosts joint-supporting vitamins and minerals.

2. Skin Allergies

Skin allergies can cause itching, scratching, and discomfort for many dogs. Including **omega-3-rich foods** and **anti-inflammatory ingredients** can help soothe the skin and promote a healthy coat.

Recipe 1: Salmon & Sweet Potato Mix

Ingredients:

- 1 cup salmon, boneless and raw if possible (cooked if preferred)
- ½ cup sweet potatoes, mashed (optional to bake lightly)
- 1 tablespoon coconut oil
- 1 small portion (approx. 1 teaspoon) raw liver or kidney (optional)

Instructions:

Mix the raw or cooked salmon with mashed sweet potatoes, then stir in coconut oil. Optional raw offal, such as liver or kidney, provides extra vitamins A and B. Salmon is rich in omega-3 fatty acids, which help soothe irritated skin, and coconut oil adds moisturizing, anti-inflammatory benefits.

Recipe 2: Duck & Quinoa Bowl

Ingredients:

- 1 cup ground duck (or raw turkey as an alternative if preferred)
- ½ cup cooked quinoa (cool before mixing)
- ¼ cup zucchini, chopped (optional to lightly steam)
- 1 tablespoon flaxseed oil
- 1 small portion (approx. 1-2 teaspoons) raw liver (optional for added nutrients)

Instructions:

Combine raw or lightly cooked ground duck with zucchini and cooked quinoa. Drizzle with flaxseed oil before serving. Duck serves as a novel protein that may reduce allergic reactions, while flaxseed oil supports skin health with omega-3s. Optional offal adds beneficial vitamins and minerals to further support skin resilience and overall health.

---

3. Weight Management

Helping your dog lose weight can be a challenge, but a balanced diet focusing on **lean proteins**, **low-fat foods**, and plenty of fibre can help them shed pounds while feeling full and satisfied.

Recipe 1: Turkey & Carrot Mix

Ingredients:

- 1 cup lean ground turkey (raw or lightly cooked)
- ½ cup shredded carrots
- ¼ cup green beans, chopped (optional to steam lightly)
- 1 teaspoon coconut oil (use sparingly to keep the meal low-fat)
- 1 small portion (approx. 1 teaspoon) raw liver or kidney (optional for nutrient boost)

Instructions:

Combine raw or lightly cooked turkey with carrots, green beans, and optional raw liver or kidney. Add a small amount of coconut oil for flavour and nutrients but use sparingly to keep it low-fat. This high-fibre, low-fat meal is designed to help your dog feel full without adding extra calories.

Recipe 2: Chicken & Green Bean Dinner

Ingredients:

- 1 cup shredded chicken breast (raw or lightly cooked, skinless, boneless)
- ½ cup green beans, chopped (optional to steam lightly)
- ¼ cup pumpkin puree
- 1 small portion (approx. 1-2 teaspoons) raw liver (optional for added nutrients)

Instructions:

Mix shredded chicken breast with green beans, pumpkin puree, and optional raw liver. Pumpkin provides fibre without adding many calories, making this an ideal meal for dogs needing weight management. The optional offal boosts the meal's nutrient content while remaining lean.

4. Digestive Health

A healthy gut is key to your dog's overall well-being. If your dog has a sensitive stomach, try meals that are easily digestible and incorporate **probiotic-rich foods** to improve gut health.

Recipe 1: Pumpkin & Kefir Digestive Boost

Ingredients

- ½ cup pumpkin puree
- ¼ cup plain kefir (unsweetened, unflavoured)
- ¼ cup cooked white rice (optional for extra fibre)
- 1 small portion (approx. 1 teaspoon) raw liver or kidney (optional for digestive support)

Instructions:

Combine the pumpkin puree and kefir in a bowl, mixing in rice and optional raw liver or kidney if desired. The probiotics in kefir support gut health, while pumpkin provides gentle fibre to aid digestion and help alleviate diarrhea or constipation. The addition of offal offers vitamins and minerals that support a balanced digestive system.

Tip: For an extra boost, rotate between liver and kidney to provide a variety of digestive-supporting nutrients.

Recipe 2: Turkey & Rice Gentle Stew

Ingredients:

- 1 cup lean ground turkey (raw or lightly cooked)
- ½ cup cooked white rice
- ¼ cup carrots, chopped (optional to steam lightly)
- 1 tablespoon plain yogurt (unsweetened, unflavoured)
- 1 small portion (approx. 1 tablespoon) raw liver or kidney (optional, finely chopped)

Instructions:

Mix the raw or lightly cooked turkey with rice, carrots, and yogurt, adding optional finely chopped raw liver or kidney to enhance nutrient content. This gentle, easily digestible meal is perfect for dogs with sensitive stomachs. Turkey provides lean protein, yogurt adds probiotics for gut health, and the offal adds key vitamins to further support digestion.

Tip: If your dog is new to offal, start with a small amount and gradually increase to ensure gentle digestion.

---

5. Urinary Health

Dogs prone to **urinary tract infections (UTIs)** or bladder issues can benefit from a diet that supports urinary health. Ingredients like **cranberries** and **antioxidant-rich foods** can help reduce the frequency of UTIs and promote a healthy bladder.

Recipe 1: Chicken & Cranberry Delight

Ingredients:

- 1 cup shredded chicken breast (skinless, boneless, raw or lightly cooked)
- ¼ cup fresh or dried cranberries (unsweetened)
- ¼ cup zucchini, chopped (optional to steam lightly)
- 1 small portion (approx. 1 teaspoon) raw kidney or liver (optional for added nutrients)

Instructions:

Mix shredded chicken with cranberries, zucchini, and optional raw liver or kidney. Cranberries support urinary tract health by helping to prevent bacteria from adhering to bladder walls, while the addition of offal enhances the meal with vitamins that promote immune and organ health.

Tip: Rotate between fresh and dried cranberries to add variety and start with small portions of offal to introduce new flavours gently.

Recipe 2: Beef & Blueberry Medley

Ingredients:

- 1 cup lean ground beef (raw or lightly cooked if preferred)
- ¼ cup fresh blueberries
- ½ cup green beans, chopped (optional to steam lightly)
- 1 small portion (approx. 1-2 teaspoons) raw kidney (optional for extra nutrients)

Instructions:

Combine raw or lightly cooked ground beef with green beans and blueberries, adding optional raw kidney for additional vitamins. Blueberries are rich in antioxidants that support urinary and immune health, while lean beef provides protein without excess fat. The offal option adds iron and B vitamins, further enhancing overall well-being.

Tip: For variety, consider alternating between blueberries and cranberries as antioxidant-rich additions to support urinary health.

Conclusion: Customizing for Health

By adjusting your dog's diet to meet their specific health needs, you're not only improving their quality of life but also giving them the tools they need to thrive. The recipes above offer variety, so your dog can enjoy a healthy, balanced diet that targets their specific condition, whether it's joint health, skin issues, weight management, or digestive concerns.

Always consult your veterinarian before making significant changes to your dog's diet, especially if they have pre-existing health conditions.

What's Next?

From here, you can explore more delicious treats in the **Bonus Recipe Section** or begin the **30-Day Transition to Nutrition Challenge** for a step-by-step guide to improving your dog's overall health.

Chapter Three

Hydration and Its Importance

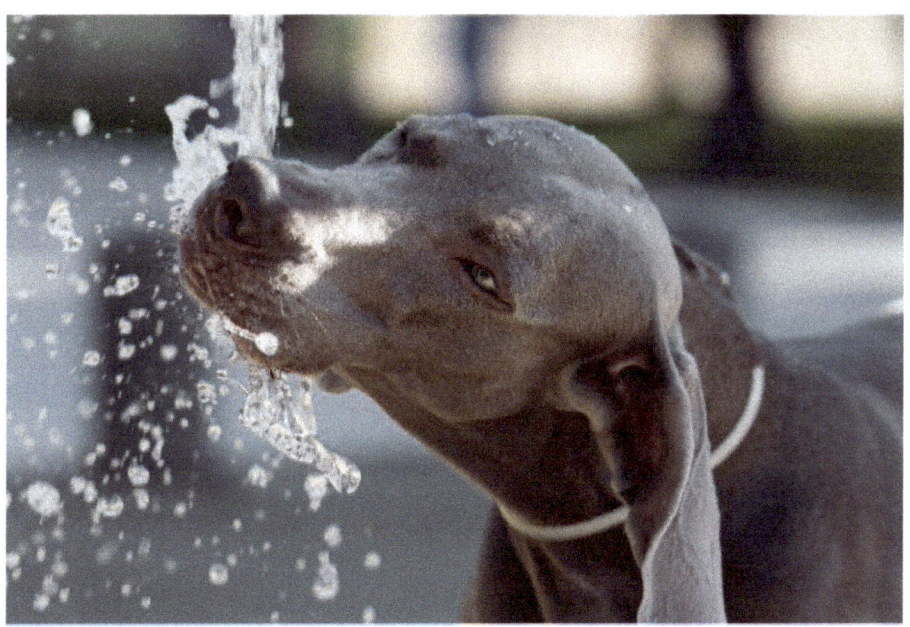

Introduction: Water—The Lifeblood of Your Dog's Health

Water is one of the most critical nutrients for your dog's health, yet it's often overlooked in discussions about nutrition. Hydration isn't just about quenching thirst—it's vital for every function in your dog's body. Proper hydration ensures that your dog's joints stay lubricated, their organs function optimally, and toxins are flushed from their system.

But not all water sources are equal. Tap water, for example, can contain chemicals like fluoride and chlorine, which can lead to toxic overload over time. Whenever possible, opt for **clean, filtered water** to avoid exposing your dog to unnecessary toxins.

In this chapter, we'll explore the importance of hydration, signs of dehydration, and how you can keep your dog hydrated in healthy ways—even when it's hot outside.

---

1. Clean Water vs. Tap Water: Why It Matters

While most of us provide tap water to our dogs, it's worth noting that tap water can contain harmful chemicals such as:

- **Chlorine**
- **Fluoride**
- **Heavy metals** (like lead or copper)

These chemicals are often added to tap water to make it safe for human consumption, but they aren't always ideal for dogs. Long-term exposure to certain chemicals can contribute to health problems like skin irritations, digestive issues, and even toxic buildup in the organs.

Whenever possible, provide your dog with **filtered or distilled water**. This minimizes their exposure to chemicals and ensures they stay hydrated with the purest water available.

---

2. Signs of Dehydration in Dogs

It's essential to monitor your dog for signs of dehydration, especially during the summer months or after periods of intense exercise. Common signs of dehydration include:

- **Excessive panting**
- **Dry gums or nose**
- **Lethargy**
- **Loss of skin elasticity** (If you gently lift the skin on the back of your dog's neck and it doesn't quickly snap back into place, they may be dehydrated.)
- **Sunken eyes**
- **Dark urine** or decreased urination

If your dog is showing signs of dehydration, you need to act fast. Offer clean water, and if they refuse to drink, try adding a little low-sodium bone broth to their water to encourage them. In severe cases of dehydration, a visit to the vet may be necessary for IV fluids.

---

3. Hydrating Foods: Boosting Water Intake Through Diet

While water is the primary way to keep your dog hydrated, certain foods can also help. Hydrating foods naturally contain high water content and can be added to your dog's diet to help them stay hydrated, especially during the hotter months.

Key Hydrating Foods:

- **Cucumber**: 95% water and a great crunchy treat.
- **Watermelon**: Low in calories and made up of 92% water (just avoid the seeds and rind).

- **Bone Broth**: Rich in nutrients and hydrating—serve it cold on a hot day for a refreshing treat.
- **Zucchini**: Packed with water and easily added to meals.
- **Celery**: 95% water and a good source of fibre.
- **Pumpkin**: While not as high in water content, it helps with digestion and keeps things moving, which is important for overall hydration.

Incorporating these foods into your dog's meals or as snacks can provide an extra hydration boost, especially if your dog is reluctant to drink water.

---

4. Hydration in Hot Weather: Keeping Your Dog Cool

During summer or after exercise, keeping your dog cool and hydrated is crucial. Dogs lose a lot of water through panting, so ensuring they stay hydrated during these times is important.

Tips for Keeping Your Dog Hydrated in Hot Weather:

- **Frozen Treats**: Offer your dog frozen bone broth or ice cubes made from low-sodium chicken broth. You can also make icy treats using hydrating fruits like watermelon or cucumber.
- **Shade and Fresh Water**: Always provide access to shade and a constant supply of fresh, clean water when your dog is outdoors. Consider using a cooling mat or letting your dog paddle in shallow water to lower their body temperature.

- **Limit Exercise in Heat**: Reduce exercise during the hottest parts of the day. Take your dog for walks early in the morning or later in the evening when it's cooler.
- **Offer Small, Frequent Drinks**: If your dog has been exercising or is out in the sun, offer small amounts of water frequently, rather than letting them gulp down large quantities at once, which could upset their stomach.

5. Hydration and Nutrition: The Connection

It's important to understand that hydration goes beyond just water intake. Proper hydration helps the body digest food, regulate temperature, and eliminate waste. When dogs are dehydrated, they can experience **digestive issues**, **urinary tract problems**, and even **kidney stress**.

A diet rich in **moist, whole foods** (like the hydrating vegetables and fruits mentioned earlier) supports hydration and makes it easier for dogs to digest their food. If your dog eats a lot of dry kibble, make sure to always have plenty of water available, as kibble can contribute to dehydration if not balanced with adequate water intake.

Conclusion: Hydration for a Healthy Dog

Hydration is the cornerstone of your dog's overall health. Keeping them well-hydrated with **clean, fresh water** and hydrating foods not only improves their energy and digestion but also supports every major bodily function. During hotter months, or if your dog is particularly active, hydration becomes even more critical.

By providing your dog with **pure water** and a diet rich in hydrating foods, you're ensuring that they stay healthy, comfortable, and full of energy all year round.

Chapter 4
Monitoring Your Dog's Health Through Diet

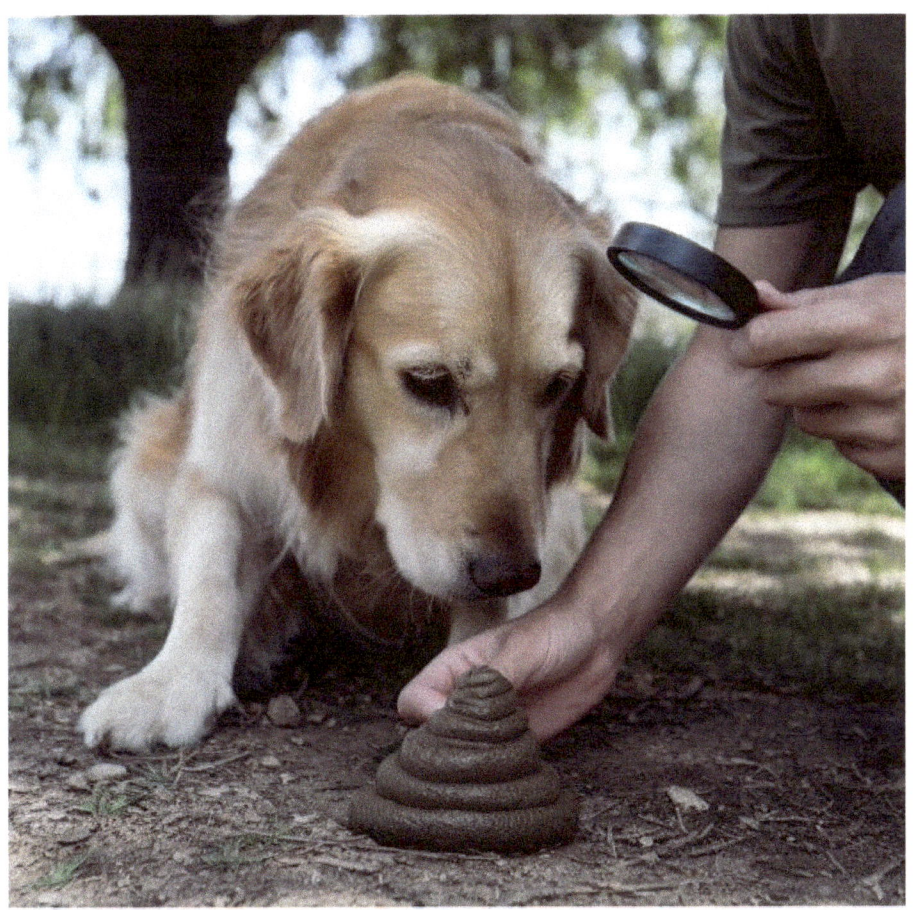

Why Monitoring Your Dog's Health Matters

When it comes to our dogs, we often notice changes in their health through their behaviour, coat, or energy levels. But did you know that your dog's **diet** is at the core of these signals? Just like children, certain ingredients in food can impact not only your dog's health but also their **behaviour** and **emotions**.

One of the most essential, yet often overlooked, ways to monitor your dog's health is by paying attention to their **stool**—or as we more commonly call it, **poo**. Yep, we're talking about poop. No one really loves discussing it, but the truth is, your dog's poop is a window into their overall health. And believe it or not, it can tell you a lot more than you think!

By observing their poop (yes, poop!), you can learn about how their diet is affecting them physically, and even emotionally. Let's dive into the signs that will help you understand what their poop (and more) is telling you.

Poo Quality: What It Tells You About Their Diet and Emotions

Okay, so poop. We might joke about it, but it's one of the best indicators of your dog's digestive and overall health. A healthy poop is a sign that things are going well, while loose, dry, or discoloured poo can point to dietary or emotional issues. And, yes, just like us, dogs can have tummy troubles when they're stressed or anxious, which often shows up as runny poo. So it's not just about what they eat, but also how they feel.

What to Look For:

- **Healthy Stool** (a.k.a. poop!): Firm but not hard, moist but not watery, and easy to pick up. If you're able to scoop it without cringing, you're on the right track! The colour should be a medium brown.
- **Loose or Runny Poo**: If your dog's poop is watery or loose, it could mean their diet is too rich in fat or fibre, or they might be reacting to something new in their food. But it's not just about diet—dogs, like us, can have digestive upset when they're feeling anxious. So if they're stressed, you might see runnier poo.
- **Dry, Hard Poo**: On the flip side, dry, crumbly poop can mean your dog isn't getting enough hydration or fibre. Make sure they're drinking enough water and consider adding hydrating foods like broth or veggies to their diet to soften things up.
- **Discoloured Poop**: Black, yellow, or green poop can be a sign of something more serious. If you notice these colours, it's best to check in with your vet to make sure everything's okay.

So, while poop might not be your favourite topic, it's an essential one! By regularly checking your dog's poo, you can catch signs of digestive or emotional issues early and make the necessary diet adjustments to keep them healthy.

Coat & Skin: A Reflection of Nutrition and Emotional Well-being

Your dog's **coat and skin** are direct indicators of their overall health and nutrition, but they can also reflect their emotional state. A dog who is stressed, anxious, or unsettled may show signs of this in their skin and coat, such as excessive shedding or dullness. Nutritionally, a lack of **essential fats** or hidden allergens in their food can contribute to skin issues, but emotional factors can play a role as well.

What to Look For:

- **Shiny, Soft Coat**: A healthy coat should feel soft and look shiny, often indicating that your dog is getting enough essential fatty acids, especially omega-3s and omega-6s, found in fish oil, flaxseed, and high-quality proteins.
- **Dry, Flaky Skin**: This can be a sign that your dog isn't getting enough healthy fats in their diet, or they may be dealing with a food allergy. However, it can also be stress related. Dogs who are anxious may scratch or lick themselves more frequently, leading to irritated skin.
- **Excessive Shedding**: While dogs naturally shed, excessive shedding can sometimes indicate poor nutrition or an allergy. In some cases, stress or anxiety can trigger excessive shedding as well, so it's worth considering both physical and emotional factors if you notice this change.

By keeping an eye on your dog's coat, skin, and behaviour, you can identify not only nutritional gaps but also emotional stressors that may be affecting their health.

Energy Levels: A Sign of Balanced Nutrition and Emotional Health

A dog's **energy levels** are one of the easiest ways to spot whether their diet is doing its job, but they're also tied to emotional well-being. Dogs who are stressed, anxious, or even bored may exhibit changes in their energy. A well-fed dog with a balanced diet and a healthy emotional state should have **steady energy** throughout the day, without sudden spikes or crashes.

What to Look For:

- **Steady Energy**: If your dog seems content and active without being overly hyper, it's a good sign their diet is balanced. This shows they're getting the right combination of **protein**, **fats**, and **carbohydrates**. Emotionally, a calm and balanced dog will often have steady energy levels, too.
- **Lethargy**: If your dog seems sluggish or uninterested in activities they usually enjoy, it could be a sign that their diet isn't providing enough energy. Emotional factors like sadness, boredom, or anxiety can also contribute to low energy levels.
- **Hyperactivity**: Dogs that are overly hyper may be consuming too many simple carbohydrates (like those found in processed kibble) or they may be reacting to food additives. Emotional triggers, like excitement, fear, or overstimulation, can also lead to hyperactive behaviour. Switching to a diet that's higher in protein and healthy fats can help balance their energy levels, while providing a stable, calming environment can reduce hyperactivity.

By paying attention to any sudden changes in your dog's energy levels, you can determine whether their diet or emotional health may be the cause.

When to Adjust Your Dog's Diet

If you notice any of the signs above—whether it's changes in poop, coat, energy, or behaviour—it might be time to make adjustments to your dog's diet. Here's how to approach dietary changes:

Gradual Changes:

When making any changes to your dog's diet, it's important to do so **gradually**. Sudden shifts can cause digestive upset, so introduce new foods or adjust portion sizes over a period of **7-10 days**. Start by mixing a small amount of the new food with their current food and slowly increase the ratio.

Focus on High-Quality Proteins:

If your dog's coat or energy levels are lacking, consider upgrading the quality of protein in their meals. Opt for **lean meats** like chicken, turkey, beef, or lamb, and rotate proteins to give them a variety of nutrients.

Increase Healthy Fats:

If their coat or skin looks dry, or if they seem low on energy, increasing **healthy fats** in their diet can make a big difference. Fish oil, flaxseed oil, and coconut oil are great additions to help with skin and coat health, as well as joint support.

Hydration:

Don't forget the importance of hydration! Ensure your dog is getting enough **clean, fresh water** each day and consider adding hydrating foods like cucumbers, watermelon, and low-sodium broths to their meals.

What Your Dog's Body and Behaviour Are Telling You

At the end of the day, your dog's body—and yes, their poop—are always communicating with you. Whether it's through their stools (ahem, poop), coat, skin, energy levels, or even their emotions, these signs offer valuable insights into how their diet—and their emotional environment—is affecting their health. By paying attention to these subtle changes, you can make the necessary adjustments to ensure your dog stays happy, healthy, and full of life.

Chapter 5

Saving on Vet Bills—How a Natural Diet Keeps Your Dog Healthy

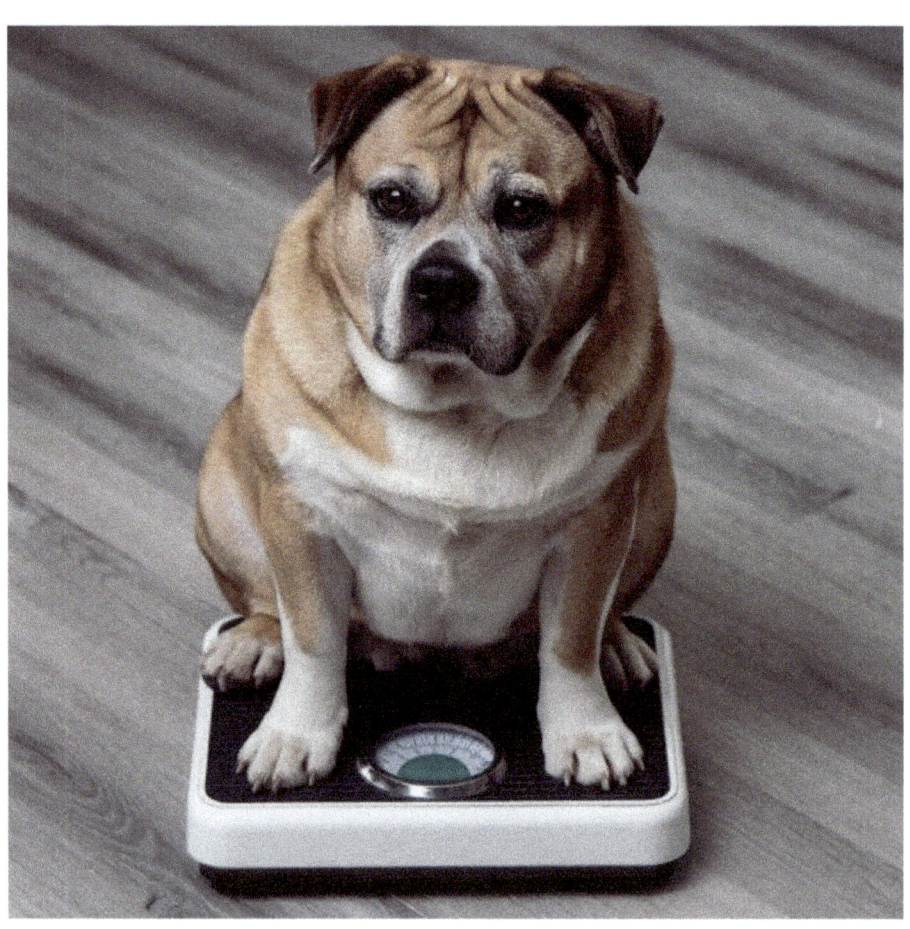

The Hidden Cost of Commercial Dog Food

At first glance, commercial dog food—especially kibble—seems like a cost-effective choice. It's easy to buy in bulk, and many brands are marketed as "complete nutrition." But the truth is, this convenience often comes at a hidden cost—**your dog's health**.

Processed pet food is often filled with low-quality ingredients, additives, and preservatives that do more harm than good in the long run. Cheap fillers, artificial colours, and synthetic vitamins may keep your dog alive, but they won't help them thrive. Over time, these ingredients can contribute to **chronic health issues** like obesity, diabetes, allergies, and joint pain—all of which can lead to frequent and expensive vet visits.

Here's the bottom line: what you save on dog food today could end up costing you **thousands** in vet bills down the road.

How a Natural Diet Prevents Common Health Problems

The good news is that by feeding your dog a **natural diet**, you can help prevent many of the most common health problems that drive people to the vet. Here's how feeding real, whole foods can keep your dog healthy and out of the vet's office:

---

1. Allergies & Skin Conditions

Many commercial dog foods contain common allergens like **corn**, **wheat**, **soy**, and artificial additives that can trigger skin problems, itching, and digestive upset in sensitive dogs. Even some vet-recommended brands use these ingredients.

Switching to a natural diet made from high-quality proteins, vegetables, and healthy fats can often eliminate these allergens and soothe your dog's skin. Foods like **fish oil**, **coconut oil**, and **novel proteins** like **duck** or **venison** are particularly good for dogs with allergies.

---

2. Joint Health & Mobility

As dogs age, they often develop **joint issues** or **arthritis**, especially larger breeds. While joint supplements and medications can help, the food you're feeding your dog plays a huge role in supporting their mobility and reducing inflammation.

A diet rich in **omega-3 fatty acids** (from fish oil or flaxseed oil), **glucosamine**, and **chondroitin** (found naturally in bone broth) can keep your dog's joints healthy and delay the need for expensive medications.

---

3. Digestive Health

Many dogs struggle with digestive issues like diarrhea, constipation, or frequent gas—often caused by the low-quality fillers and artificial ingredients in commercial pet food. Feeding your dog a natural diet full of easily digestible foods like **pumpkin**, **sweet potatoes**, and high-quality meats can help improve their digestion. **Probiotics** and **fibre-rich vegetables** can also keep your dog's gut healthy, reducing the risk of gastrointestinal issues that lead to costly vet visits.

4. Weight Management

Pet obesity is a growing problem, and it's no surprise when you look at what goes into most commercial dog foods. Many kibbles are packed with **empty calories** from grains and fillers that don't provide the nutrients your dog needs to stay at a healthy weight. Over time, obesity can lead to diabetes, heart disease, and joint pain—conditions that require long-term management and medication.

A natural diet, on the other hand, is full of **nutrient-dense** foods that help your dog feel satisfied while maintaining a healthy weight. Lean meats, vegetables, and healthy fats keep them trim without unnecessary calories, reducing the risk of obesity-related health problems.

5. Dental Health

Poor dental health is another common issue in dogs fed on processed kibble. Despite marketing claims, kibble doesn't clean your dog's teeth—it often sticks to them, promoting plaque buildup and eventually leading to gum disease, tooth loss, or costly dental surgeries.

Feeding raw bones, **chewing-friendly foods**, and incorporating natural teeth-cleaning elements like **raw meaty bones** or **carrots** can help maintain your dog's dental health, saving you from those expensive trips to the vet for dental work.

Investing in Real Food for Long-Term Savings

It's easy to get caught up in the convenience of kibble or canned food, especially when the price tag seems lower. But when you start adding up the long-term costs of treating health issues that arise from poor nutrition—vet visits, medications, supplements, even surgeries—you'll see that investing in **real food** for your dog is a much smarter choice.

By feeding your dog a **whole-food, natural diet**, you're giving them the best chance at avoiding chronic diseases and health issues. You'll likely notice fewer trips to the vet, fewer medications, and a happier, healthier dog.

The Long-Term Benefits of a Natural Diet

- **Fewer Vet Visits**: A well-fed dog with balanced nutrition is less likely to suffer from recurring health problems, saving you on vet consultations, treatments, and medications.
- **Less Need for Medications**: Many common dog health problems can be treated or prevented through diet. Fewer medications mean less stress for your dog and more money saved.
- **Improved Quality of Life**: Dogs fed a natural diet tend to live longer, healthier lives with more energy, better mobility, and fewer health complications as they age.

- **Savings on Pet Insurance**: With fewer health problems, your dog may qualify for lower pet insurance premiums, or you may need less coverage in the first place.

Why Natural Nutrition is an Investment in Your Dog's Future

Think of your dog's food as an **investment** in their future. When you choose to feed them high-quality, natural foods, you're not only giving them a better life, but you're also saving yourself from the potential costs of treating avoidable health problems. It's about **prevention over cure**—keeping your dog healthy from the inside out, rather than relying on treatments after the fact.

And let's be honest—seeing your dog happy, active, and pain-free is worth so much more than any vet bill. By investing in real nutrition today, you're making sure that your dog can enjoy life to the fullest for as long as possible.

Chapter 6

Putting It All Together—Recipes for Every Life Stage and Condition

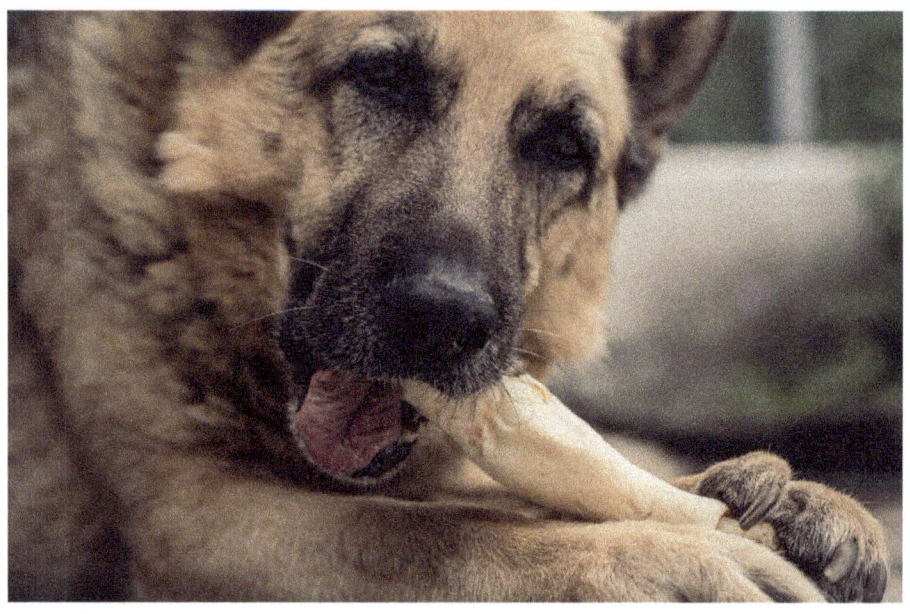

Introduction: Tailoring Your Dog's Diet

Throughout this book, we've covered the benefits of feeding your dog a natural diet and how it can support their health at every stage of life. From puppies to seniors, and for dogs with specific health conditions, a balanced, whole-food diet can make all the difference. In this chapter, we'll recap key recipes and provide practical tips on how to customize meals for your dog's age, health, and lifestyle.

Whether you're just starting with a natural diet or looking for ways to improve your dog's nutrition, this section will be your go-to resource for creating balanced, nutritious meals.

Puppies: Recipes for Growing Pups

Puppies are in a critical growth stage and need nutrient-dense meals rich in **protein**, **healthy fats**, and **calcium** to support their development. Here are some of the key recipes for puppies:

Key Puppy Recipes

1. **Raw Chicken & Veggie Mash**
   Packed with protein, essential vitamins, and nutrients for growing muscles and bones. The addition of liver provides vitamin A and other key nutrients for immune support.
2. **Baked Turkey & Pumpkin Meatballs**
   Wholesome, grain-free meatballs packed with protein and healthy fats. Optionally include ground eggshell for additional calcium to support bone growth.
3. **Frozen Salmon & Sweet Potato Cubes**
   A cooling, omega-3-rich treat perfect for teething puppies or as a summertime snack.

Customising Puppy Meals

- **Calcium**: Include bone meal or ground eggshells in small amounts to provide bioavailable calcium for bone development.

- **Protein Variety**: Rotate different proteins like chicken, turkey, and fish to ensure puppies get a range of amino acids and nutrients for well-rounded growth.
- **Small Portions**: Feed multiple small meals throughout the day to match your puppy's rapid metabolism.

Adult Dogs: Recipes for Maintenance and Energy

Adult dogs need balanced nutrition to **maintain energy levels, support muscle mass**, and **keep their coat and skin healthy**. These recipes are designed to provide the nutrients adult dogs need to stay strong, active, and happy.

Key Adult Dog Recipes

1. **Beef & Sweet Potato Bowl**
   A hearty meal filled with protein and fibre to support energy and digestive health.
2. **Raw Lamb & Veggie Patties**
   Nutrient-dense patties packed with healthy fats and protein.
3. **Chicken & Sardine Bowl**
   High in omega-3s and protein, perfect for skin and coat health.

Customizing Adult Dog Meals:

- **Protein-Rich Meals**: Focus on lean meats to maintain muscle mass and provide sustained energy.
- **Add Veggies**: Include a variety of vegetables for fibre and micronutrients.

- **Healthy Fats**: Incorporate healthy fats like fish oil or flaxseed oil to support skin, coat, and joint health.

Senior Dogs: Recipes for Joint Health and Digestion

As dogs age, their metabolism slows, and they may need meals that are easier to digest and support **joint health**. Senior dogs benefit from foods rich in **omega-3 fatty acids**, **bone broth**, and **anti-inflammatory ingredients**.

Key Senior Dog Recipes:

1. **Chicken & Bone Broth Soup**
    - A nourishing meal that supports joint health and is easy to digest.
2. **Moist Turkey & Pumpkin Loaf**
    - Soft and gentle on the stomach, with added pumpkin to aid digestion.
3. **Fish & Veggie Mix**
    - A simple, high-protein meal that's gentle on the digestive system, with added fish oil for joint health.

Customizing Senior Dog Meals:

- **Joint Support**: Add glucosamine or chondroitin supplements to support aging joints.
- **Easier to Chew**: Offer soft or easily digestible foods, especially for dogs with dental issues.
- **Smaller Portions**: Feed smaller, more frequent meals to avoid digestive upset.

Recipes for Specific Health Conditions

Dogs with specific health needs require customized diets that target those issues while providing balanced nutrition. Here are key recipes tailored to common health problems like **allergies, weight management, joint health**, and **digestive health**.

Joint Health & Arthritis:

1. **Bone Broth & Chicken Bowl**
   - Rich in glucosamine and chondroitin to support joint mobility.
2. **Salmon & Veggie Joint Boost**
   - High in omega-3s, perfect for reducing inflammation in aging joints.

Skin Allergies:

1. **Duck & Sweet Potato Pâté**
   - Free from common allergens like chicken and beef, with added coconut oil for skin health.
2. **Sardine & Coconut Oil Skin Support**
   - A simple, omega-rich meal that soothes irritated skin and reduces inflammation.

Weight Management:

1. **Low-Calorie Turkey & Carrot Mix**
   - Lean and filling, perfect for dogs needing to manage their weight.
2. **Beef & Rice Power Bowl**
   - High in protein but low in calories, with added fibre to keep dogs feeling full longer.

Digestive Health:

1. **Pumpkin & Kefir Digestive Smoothie**
   - Filled with probiotics and fibre to support gut health and regular digestion.
2. **Chicken & Oatmeal Digestive Boost**
   - A gentle, fibre-rich meal that soothes the digestive system.

How to Customize Meals for Your Dog's Needs

Every dog is different, and their diet should reflect their **age**, **health**, and **activity level**. Here are a few tips for adjusting meals to fit your dog's specific needs:

1. **Rotate Proteins**: Switching up the proteins in your dog's meals—like chicken, beef, lamb, or fish—ensures they get a variety of amino acids and nutrients. This also reduces the risk of developing sensitivities.
2. **Incorporate Supplements**: Depending on your dog's needs, you can easily add natural supplements like **fish oil** for joint health, **bone broth** for mobility, or **pumpkin** for digestion.
3. **Adjust Portions**: Make sure you're feeding the right amount for your dog's size, age, and activity level. Puppies and active adult dogs need more calories, while seniors or less active dogs benefit from smaller, more frequent meals.
4. **Hydration Matters**: Don't forget to provide **clean, fresh water** throughout the day, and consider adding hydrating foods like bone broth or cucumber to their meals to ensure they stay hydrated.

Conclusion: Putting It All Into Practice

Feeding your dog a natural, whole-food diet is one of the best things you can do to support their health at every stage of life. Whether you're feeding a growing puppy, a busy adult dog, or an aging senior, these recipes and tips will help ensure they get the nutrients they need to thrive.

Remember, it's not about perfection—it's about making small, meaningful changes that have a big impact on your dog's well-being. By focusing on high-quality ingredients, rotating proteins, and addressing specific health needs, you can create meals that are not only healthy but also delicious for your dog.

In the following **Bonus Recipe Section**, you'll find additional treat ideas to round out your dog's natural diet, ensuring they get plenty of variety, fun, and nutrition in every bite.

Chapter Seven

Bonus Recipe Section

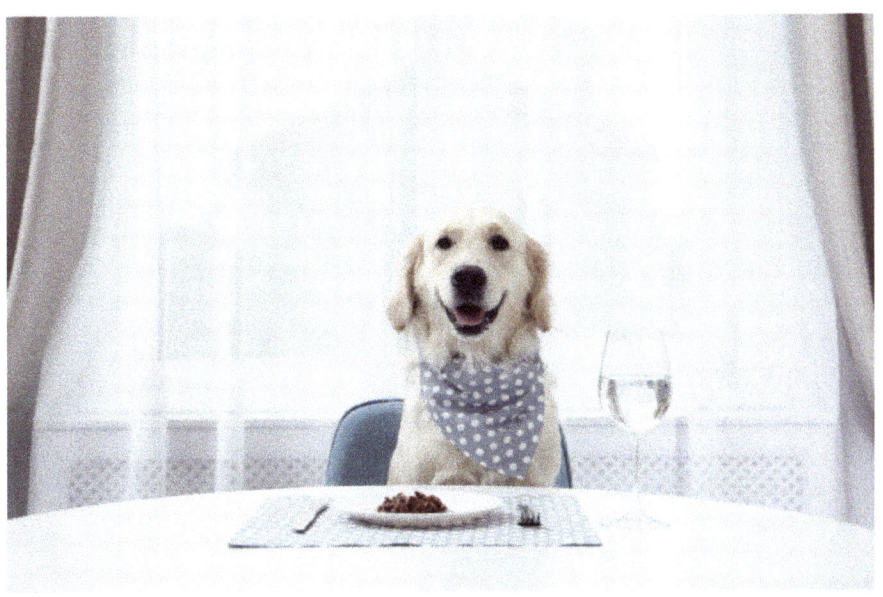

Treats and Snacks for Every Occasion

When (and Why) to Give Treats

Treats are more than just a way to show your dog some extra love—they're great for **training**, **rewarding good behaviour**, and even just bonding time. The key is to give treats in moderation and ensure they're healthy, so you know exactly what's going into your dog's body. Whether you're using treats to reinforce good behaviour on a walk or celebrating your dog's birthday, it's best to opt for **natural, homemade treats** so you can avoid the artificial junk found in many store-bought snacks.

How Often Should You Give Treats?

The general rule is that treats should make up **no more than 10%** of your dog's daily calories. This keeps their overall diet balanced while still giving them the joy of a tasty snack. Use treats strategically for training, rewarding good behaviour, or just because they deserve a little something extra. With that said, let's jump into some **deliciously natural recipes** that are fun to make—and even more fun to give!

The Classic: Peanut Butter & Pumpkin Bites

Dogs love peanut butter, and when you mix it with pumpkin, it's a match made in heaven! These treats are perfect for stuffing in your pocket during walks.

- **Ingredients**:
    - ½ cup peanut butter (natural, no added sugar or salt)
    - 1 cup pumpkin puree (unsweetened)
    - 1 ½ cups oat flour
    - 1 teaspoon cinnamon (optional)
- **Instructions**:
    1. Preheat oven to 180°C (350°F).
    2. Mix the peanut butter and pumpkin puree in a bowl.
    3. Slowly add oat flour until a dough forms.
    4. Roll out the dough and cut into shapes or use silicone moulds.
    5. Bake for 15-20 minutes until firm.
    6. Let cool before serving.

Pro tip: These are great for training because they don't crumble in your pocket!

French Flair: "Biscuits pour Bouldogues Français"

In honour of French Bulldogs, here's a chic treat inspired by French cuisine. With simple ingredients and an air of elegance, these crunchy bites will have your dog saying "merci!"

- **Ingredients**:
    - ½ cup grated Parmesan cheese
    - 1 cup oat flour
    - 2 tablespoons olive oil
    - 1 egg
    - 1 teaspoon chopped parsley
- **Instructions**:
    1. Preheat oven to 180°C (350°F).
    2. Combine all ingredients and mix into a dough.
    3. Roll into small balls and flatten slightly with a fork.
    4. Bake for 15-18 minutes until golden.
    5. Let cool before serving.

Fun fact: French Bulldogs, though stylish, are still dogs. They'll roll in dirt and then beg for these treats—classic French mischief!

Frozen Fruity Pup Pops (Icy Treats for Summer)

Perfect for hot summer days, these icy treats will keep your dog cool and hydrated.

- **Ingredients**:

- 1 cup plain yogurt (unsweetened)
- ½ cup strawberries (pureed)
- ½ cup blueberries (whole)
- 1 tablespoon honey (optional)
- **Instructions**:
    1. Mix the yogurt, pureed strawberries, and honey (if using).
    2. Pour into silicone moulds, adding a blueberry or two into each mould.
    3. Freeze for at least 4 hours.
    4. Pop out and serve on a hot day!

Dog-approved bonus: Humans will love these too. Just swap the silicone mould for a popsicle tray!

"Trim & Slim" Weight Loss Treats

For dogs who need to shed a few pounds, these treats are low-calorie but still packed with flavour.

- **Ingredients**:
    - ½ cup grated zucchini
    - ½ cup grated carrots
    - 1 cup oat flour
    - 1 egg
    - 1 tablespoon coconut oil
- **Instructions**:
    1. Preheat oven to 180°C (350°F).
    2. Mix the zucchini, carrots, and coconut oil in a bowl.
    3. Stir in oat flour and the egg until a dough forms.
    4. Roll into small balls and bake for 15-20 minutes.

5. Cool before serving.

Weight-loss tip: These treats are high in fibre and low in calories, perfect for keeping your dog's weight in check without sacrificing flavour.

Moist Meat Muffins (Great for Older Dogs)

Older dogs with sensitive teeth will appreciate these soft, meaty muffins that are easy to chew but still full of flavour.

- **Ingredients**:
    - 200g ground turkey
    - 1 cup pumpkin puree
    - 1 egg
    - ½ cup rolled oats
    - 1 teaspoon turmeric (for joint health)
- **Instructions**:
    1. Preheat oven to 180°C (350°F).
    2. Mix all ingredients in a bowl until combined.
    3. Spoon the mixture into a silicone muffin tray.
    4. Bake for 25-30 minutes until cooked through.
    5. Cool and store in the fridge.

Bonus: These muffins smell so good, you'll be tempted to try one yourself (and honestly, you probably could!).

Pup-friendly Birthday Cake

Celebrate your dog's birthday with this fun and healthy birthday cake recipe. It's perfect for spoiling your dog on their special day!

- **Ingredients**:
  - 1 cup oat flour
  - ½ cup peanut butter (natural)
  - ½ cup pumpkin puree
  - 2 eggs
  - 1 teaspoon baking powder
- **For Frosting**:
  - ½ cup plain yogurt
  - 2 tablespoons peanut butter
- **Instructions**:
  1. Preheat oven to 180°C (350°F).
  2. Mix the oat flour, peanut butter, pumpkin puree, eggs, and baking powder.
  3. Pour the batter into a small cake pan and bake for 25-30 minutes.
  4. Let the cake cool before adding the yogurt-peanut butter frosting.
  5. Serve in slices!

Birthday Tip: Don't forget to add some doggie candles (just for the photos, of course!) and let your pup feel like royalty for the day.

Halloween Treats: Pumpkin & Apple Ghosts

Get into the spooky spirit with these Halloween-themed treats that are packed with fall flavours.

- **Ingredients**:
  - 1 cup pumpkin puree
  - ½ cup unsweetened applesauce
  - 1 ½ cups oat flour
  - 1 teaspoon cinnamon
- **Instructions**:

1. Preheat oven to 180°C (350°F).
2. Mix the pumpkin puree and applesauce.
3. Add the oat flour and cinnamon to form a dough.
4. Roll out and cut into ghost shapes (or any fun Halloween shape!).
5. Bake for 15-18 minutes until firm.
6. Let cool before serving.

Halloween bonus: These treats are human-friendly too. Whip up a batch for both you and your dog to enjoy during a Halloween movie marathon!

Get the Kids Involved: DIY Doggy Biscuits

Here's a fun recipe to get the whole family involved. Kids will love making these simple, fun dog biscuits, and the dogs will love eating them!

- **Ingredients**:
    - 1 cup whole wheat flour
    - ½ cup peanut butter
    - ½ cup unsweetened applesauce
    - 1 egg
- **Instructions**:
    1. Preheat oven to 180°C (350°F).
    2. Mix all ingredients together until a dough forms.
    3. Roll out the dough and use cookie cutters to create fun shapes.
    4. Bake for 15-20 minutes until golden brown.
    5. Let cool, and let the kids feed them to their furry friends!

Fun family activity: Let the kids decorate the dog biscuits with yogurt "icing" or press in some blueberries for added fun.

Final Thoughts on Treats

Giving your dog healthy, homemade treats is not only fun but also a great way to ensure they're eating nutritious, high-quality ingredients. Whether you're training, rewarding, or just showing them some extra love, these treats can be made easily at home and customized to suit your dog's needs.

Remember to source **organic** or **homegrown** ingredients when possible, and always keep the treats in balance with your dog's regular diet.

Chapter Eight

The 30-Day Transition to Nutrition Challenge

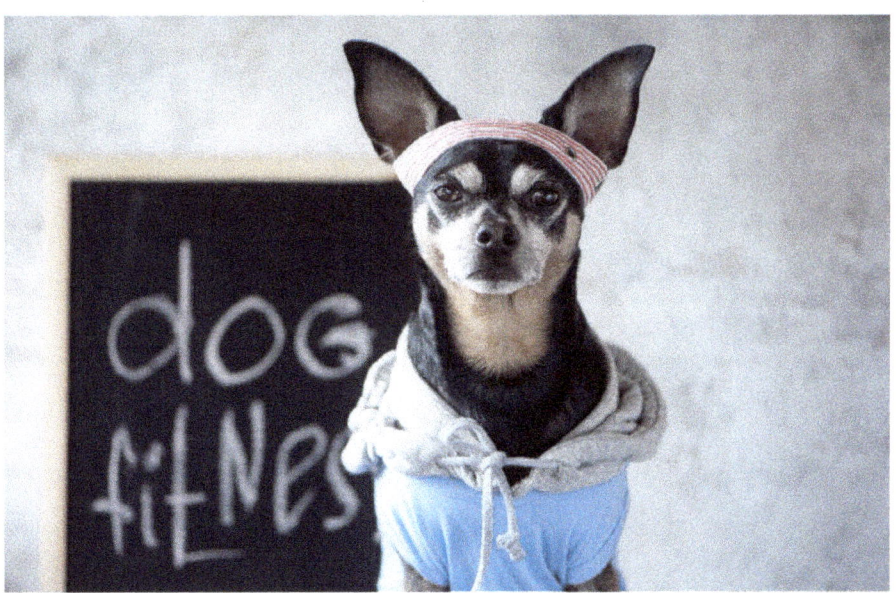

Introduction: Ready to Change Your Dog's Life?

Welcome to the **30-Day Transition to Nutrition Challenge!** Ready to see your dog thrive on a natural diet? Over the next month, we'll slowly transition your dog from processed commercial foods to wholesome, real ingredients. By the end, your dog will be **healthier**, **happier**, and, dare we say, a little more **glamorous**—shiny coat, great breath, and better poop. (Yes, even poop can be a win!)

Share your journey on social media with **#TransitionToNutrition** and tag **#MajellasPetStore** to join the community of dog lovers who are making the switch, too. Follow us on **Facebook** and **Instagram** at [Majella's Pet Store] to stay connected and see how others are progressing!

How It Works

The 30-day challenge is all about making the switch to a **natural diet** in a way that's easy on your dog's system. We'll start slow, with small changes, and work our way up to a fully homemade, natural diet by the end of the month. Along the way, keep a simple **planner or journal** to track your dog's progress—document their coat, energy levels, poop (yes, poop!), and overall health improvements.

Post your progress with **#TransitionToNutrition** and tag **#MajellasPetStore** on social media to be part of a supportive, like-minded community!

Week 1: The 25% Switch

This week, we're taking it slow—introducing natural foods into your dog's diet at **25%** of their total intake. Think of it like dipping your toes into the dog food world of gourmet goodness.

- **What to Add**: Lean meats (like chicken or beef) and some basic veggies (carrots or sweet potatoes). These are like the building blocks of a healthy diet, and trust us, your dog will be wagging their tail in excitement.
- **What to Watch For**: Keep an eye on their **poop**. Yep, we're still talking about poop. Any changes in texture are normal during the transition. Firmer, more well-formed poop means things are going well. You might also start seeing a little **extra pep in their step**—and maybe, just maybe, their breath won't knock you out anymore!
- **Goal for the Week**: By the end of Week 1, your dog should be on 25% natural food. Snap a **before photo** of your dog's coat and energy level. You'll want to look back at it later to see the transformation!

Week 2: 50% Natural Goodness

Time to crank it up! This week, we're moving to **50% natural food** and **50% their usual food**. Your dog's getting more fresh, real food, and you'll start seeing some exciting changes.

- **What to Add**: Add more variety—try **turkey**, **fish**, and **leafy greens** like spinach. Throw in some **bone broth** to support their joints (and add flavour).
- **What to Watch For**: The poop patrol continues—by now, their poop should be pretty solid and easy to pick up. Less cringing, prouder poop-scooping moments! You may also notice a bit more **shine to their coat**. And hey, if you're brave, lean in and take a whiff of their breath—you might not faint this time!

- **Goal for the Week**: Get to that 50% natural goodness and notice how your dog's energy and poop are improving. Share your halfway progress on social media, tagging **#TransitionToNutrition** and **#MajellasPetStore**!

Week 3: 75% Natural Diet

You're almost there! By Week 3, we're going for **75% natural food**, with only a small portion of their old food left. Your dog is now getting the best of the best.

- **What to Add**: Time to bring in the big guns—**organ meats** like liver and heart (your dog will LOVE these), plus more healthy fats like **fish oil** or **coconut oil** for that glossy coat.
- **What to Watch For**: This is the week where you'll really start to see the magic. Poop-wise, you're looking at a masterpiece—firm, well-formed poop that's a breeze to pick up. Their coat should be shinier, and their breath? Dare we say, it might even be tolerable!
- **Goal for the Week**: By the end of Week 3, your dog is eating 75% natural food. Their energy should be on the up, and their coat should be noticeably shinier. Share your progress with the **#TransitionToNutrition** challenge and tag **#MajellasPetStore** so we can celebrate with you!

Week 4: 100% Natural Diet

You've made it! This week, your dog's meals are **100% natural**, and the transformation should be complete. Get ready to see the results of all your hard work.

- **What to Add**: Continue with a variety of proteins, veggies, and healthy fats. Rotate ingredients to keep things interesting and balanced. Maybe treat your dog to one of those delicious homemade treats you whipped up from the **Bonus Recipe Section**!
- **What to Watch For**: By now, their poop should be **firm and perfect**—the kind of poop you don't mind picking up (okay, you probably still mind, but at least it's easier!). Their coat should be silky, their energy high, and you might even be wondering if you switched dogs.
- **Goal for the Week**: By the end of Week 4, your dog is fully transitioned to a natural diet. Take that **after photo** and admire the difference! Post it online using **#TransitionToNutrition** and tag **#MajellasPetStore** to show off your healthy, happy pup.

What to Expect After 30 Days

By the end of this challenge, here's what you can expect:

- **Poop Perfection**: Yep, that's right—firm, easy-to-pick-up poop that'll make you (almost) proud.
- **Shiny Coat**: Your dog's coat will be softer, shinier, and probably more stroke-worthy than ever before.
- **Better Breath**: You might not need to lean away when your dog gives you a slobbery kiss. Goodbye, stinky breath!

- **More Energy**: You'll see your dog bouncing around with newfound energy, ready for playtime or a good, long walk.
- **Healthier Skin**: Less itching, scratching, or signs of allergies—you may even notice a glow!
- **Improved Digestion**: With better digestion, you'll see more regular bowel movements and fewer tummy troubles.

Keeping the Momentum Going

Once you've completed the challenge, keep it up! The transition may be over, but the benefits will keep growing as your dog continues to thrive on their natural diet. Continue rotating proteins, using healthy treats, and maintaining hydration to support their overall health.

Share Your Journey!

We'd love to see your dog's transformation. Don't forget to tag us in your posts using **#TransitionToNutrition** and **#MajellasPetStore** and share your journey on **Facebook** and **Instagram** at [Majella's Pet Store]. Let's keep building a community of healthy, happy pets!

Legal Notice: Consult Your Vet

While we've designed this challenge to support a smooth transition to a natural diet, it's always a good idea to check in with your vet, especially if your dog has any pre-existing conditions or health concerns.

Call to Action

Join the Natural Dog Nutrition Revolution!

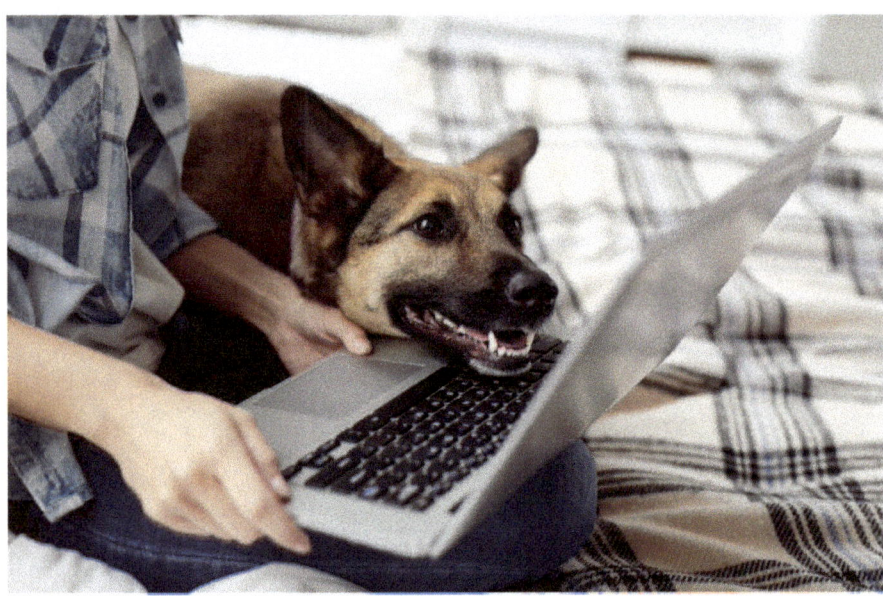

Now that you've completed the book and started your dog on their journey to better health, don't stop here! Stay connected with us and a community of passionate dog lovers who are dedicated to giving their pets the best possible life.

Here's How You Can Stay Involved:

- **Share Your Journey**: Use **#TransitionToNutrition** and **#MajellasPetStore** to show off your dog's transformation! Share photos of your dog's progress

and connect with other pet parents who are on the same journey.
- **Visit Our Website**: Head to [Majella's Pet Store](#) for informative blogs, fun products to keep your pets entertained, well-dressed, and the talk of the dog park! You'll also find exclusive tips on how to maintain your dog's health naturally.
- **Exclusive Discount**: When you visit our website, don't miss out on a **special discount** on your first order! Subscribe for weekly updates, new product launches, and the latest news on our upcoming book releases—right in your inbox!
- **Leave a Review**: If this book has made a difference in your dog's life, we'd love to hear from you! Leave a review and help other pet owners discover the benefits of a natural diet for their pets.

Glossary

Additives

Substances added to commercial dog food to enhance flavour, texture, or shelf life. Many additives, such as artificial colours and preservatives, can cause health issues in dogs over time.

BHA/BHT (Butylated Hydroxyanisole/Butylated Hydroxytoluene)

Preservatives commonly used in both human and pet foods to prevent fats from becoming rancid. Both BHA and BHT are suspected to be **carcinogens** (cancer-causing substances) and are banned in some countries, but still appear in many dog foods.

Bone Broth

A nutritious liquid made by simmering bones in water, often for long periods, to extract beneficial nutrients like **collagen**, **glucosamine**, and **chondroitin**, which help with joint health and digestion.

Carcinogen

A substance capable of causing cancer in living tissue. Many artificial additives and preservatives in commercial dog food, such as **BHA** and **ethoxyquin**, have been linked to cancer risks.

Chondroitin

A natural substance found in animal cartilage, often used to support joint health. Chondroitin helps reduce inflammation and can slow the progression of **arthritis** in dogs.

Ethoxyquin

A synthetic antioxidant used as a preservative in pet foods and some fish meals. It's a known **carcinogen** and is banned in some countries but continues to be used in many commercial dog foods.

Fillers

Low-quality ingredients added to commercial dog food to bulk up the product without providing much nutritional value. Common fillers include **corn**, **soy**, and **wheat**, which can lead to weight gain, allergies, and digestive issues.

Fish Oil

A rich source of **omega-3 fatty acids**, which help improve coat health, reduce inflammation, and support joint function. Often added to dog diets for its anti-inflammatory properties and to enhance skin and coat health.

Glucosamine

A naturally occurring compound found in **bone broth** and cartilage. It helps to build and maintain cartilage in joints, making it an excellent supplement for dogs with **arthritis** or joint pain.

Kibble

Dry dog food made from a mixture of ingredients that are baked into small, hard pieces. While convenient, kibble often contains fillers, additives, and preservatives that can lead to long-term health issues in dogs.

Novel Proteins

Proteins that are not commonly found in commercial dog food, such as **duck**, **venison**, or **kangaroo**. Novel proteins are often used in elimination diets or for dogs with allergies to more common proteins like chicken or beef.

Omega-3 Fatty Acids

Essential fatty acids found in fish oil, flaxseed, and certain meats. Omega-3s reduce inflammation, support brain function, and improve coat and skin health in dogs.

Organ Meats

Nutrient-rich meats from the organs of animals, including liver, heart, and kidney. These are high in essential vitamins (such as A, B, and iron) and minerals, supporting various health functions like immune strength, energy, and heart health. Organ meats are a beneficial component of a dog's natural diet, providing nutrients not found in muscle meats alone.

Preservatives

Chemicals added to dog food to extend shelf life. Some preservatives, like **BHA**, **BHT**, and **ethoxyquin**, have been linked to health problems like cancer and allergies.

Probiotics

Live bacteria that are beneficial for digestive health. Adding **probiotic-rich foods** like kefir or yogurt to your dog's diet can improve gut health and boost their immune system.

Raw Diet

A diet that consists of uncooked meats, bones, and vegetables, intended to mimic what dogs would eat in the wild. The raw diet focuses on providing high-quality, natural ingredients without processing or additives.

Sweet Potatoes

A starchy root vegetable that is rich in vitamins A and C, fibre, and antioxidants. Sweet potatoes are commonly used in dog food and treats for their digestive benefits and as a natural carbohydrate source.

Turmeric

A yellow spice known for its anti-inflammatory properties. Turmeric is often added to dog food for its ability to reduce inflammation, support joint health, and act as an antioxidant.

Wheat/Corn/Soy

Common **fillers** found in many commercial dog foods that provide little nutritional value. These ingredients are often linked to allergies and intolerances in dogs, leading to digestive issues, skin problems, and weight gain.

Whole Foods

Unprocessed, natural foods that are rich in nutrients. A **whole-food diet** for dogs consists of lean meats, vegetables, fruits, and healthy fats, without fillers, additives, or artificial ingredients.

Recommended Reading/Resources

For those wanting to dig deeper into the benefits of a natural diet and holistic pet care, here are some valuable books and resources:

Books:

- **"Give Your Dog a Bone"** by Dr. Ian Billinghurst
  A comprehensive guide to raw feeding and the benefits of a biologically appropriate diet for dogs.
- **"Raw and Natural Nutrition for Dogs"** by Lew Olson
  This book offers practical advice on feeding raw diets and includes recipes for every life stage.
- **"The BARF Diet"** by Dr. Ian Billinghurst
  A look into the Biologically Appropriate Raw Food (BARF) diet, focusing on the nutritional needs of dogs and the benefits of feeding raw.

Websites:

- **Dogs Naturally Magazine** (https://www.dogsnaturallymagazine.com/)
  A great resource for natural pet care, holistic treatments, and raw feeding tips.
- **Planet Paws** (https://www.planetpaws.ca/)
  Founded by Rodney Habib, Planet Paws is a leading source of information on raw diets, natural nutrition, and pet wellness.
- **Keep the Tail Wagging** (https://keepthetailwagging.com/)
  A raw feeding blog dedicated to providing information,

advice, and recipes for those looking to improve their dog's health through natural nutrition.

For more resources and tips, visit **Majella's Pet Store** at https://majellaspetstore.com/.

Conclusion

A Personal Note

As I finish writing this book, my thoughts return to why I began this journey in the first place. I have always been deeply connected to animals—whether it's a loyal dog by my side or a wild animal in need of care, they have been my motivation to keep learning, sharing, and advocating for their well-being.

Through this book, I hope to have inspired you to make conscious, informed decisions about your dog's diet and overall health. Our pets trust us to provide them with the care they deserve, and by nourishing them with real, whole foods, we honor that trust in the best way possible.

I'm not a vet or a nutritionist—I'm someone who has worked closely with animals all my life. The knowledge I share comes from experience, observation, and a deep love for animals. I've seen the impact that a proper, natural diet can have, and I believe it's within all of us to make the changes necessary for our pets' long-term health.

Thank you for taking the time to read this book. I hope you and your dog enjoy this journey together. Let's continue learning, growing, and caring for our animals with the love and respect they deserve.

With heartfelt gratitude,

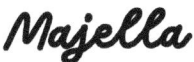

About the Author

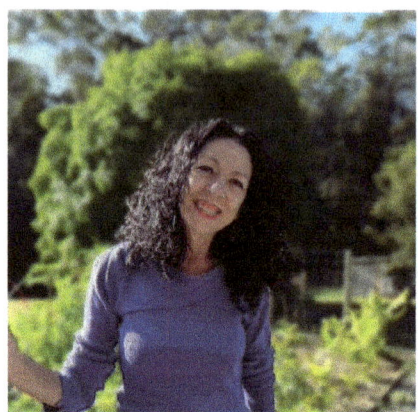

Majella Gee has spent her life working with animals, driven by a passion for their care and well-being. From her early years caring for pets and working at the local pet store to decades of experience in managing pet shops and wildlife rehabilitation, Majella's journey has always been about making a difference in the lives of animals.

Majella has become a trusted voice for pet owners, offering practical advice on natural nutrition, responsible ownership, and holistic pet care. Her work with veterinarians, animal behaviorists, and wildlife specialists has deepened her understanding of the connection between diet and health in animals.

Living in the beautiful Sunshine Coast hinterland, Majella continues to advocate for animal rights and share her knowledge through her writing. Whether through books, blogs, or one-on-one advice, Majella's goal is simple: to help more pets live long, healthy, and happy lives.

You can follow Majella's journey and find more resources at https://majellaspetstore.com/ and on social media under **#MajellasPetStore**.

Legal Notice

Title: What's Really in Your Dog's Bowl? The Essential Guide to Natural Nutrition
Author: Majella Gee
Publisher: Sorjam Publishing
ISBN: [Enter ISBN Here]

Copyright © 2024 by Majella Gee. All rights reserved.

No part of this book may be reproduced, distributed, or transmitted in any form or by any means, including photocopying, recording, or other electronic or mechanical methods, without the prior written permission of the publisher, except in the case of brief quotations embodied in critical reviews and certain other non-commercial uses permitted by copyright law. For permission requests, write to the publisher, addressed "Attention: Permissions Coordinator," at the address below.

Publisher Contact Information:
Sorjam Publishing
Email: hello@majellaspetstore.com
Website: https://majellaspetstore.com/

This book is a work of nonfiction. While the author has made every effort to ensure the accuracy and completeness of the information contained within, the advice and opinions expressed are based on personal experiences and independent research. The author and publisher assume no responsibility for errors or omissions.

Disclaimer:

The information provided in this book is for educational purposes only. It is not intended to substitute for professional veterinary advice, diagnosis, or treatment. Always seek the guidance of your veterinarian or another qualified pet care professional before making any significant changes to your dog's diet, especially if your dog has pre-existing health conditions or specific dietary needs.

The author and publisher assume no liability for any damages or injuries that may result from the use of, or reliance on, the information provided in this book. Every dog is unique, and what works for one may not work for another. Therefore, it is essential to consult a veterinarian for individual guidance and recommendations.

Veterinary care: This book is not a substitute for veterinary care. Always follow the advice of your veterinarian, especially if your dog shows signs of illness, distress, or adverse reactions to changes in their diet or environment.

Trademark Notice:

All product names, logos, and brands mentioned in this book are the property of their respective owners. All company, product, and service names used in this book are for identification purposes only. The use of these names, logos, and brands does not imply endorsement by the author or publisher.

www.ingramcontent.com/pod-product-compliance
Lightning Source LLC
Chambersburg PA
CBHW061211070526
44583CB00025B/3202